Arthritis-Pain-Remedies

Table of Contents

Introduction

Arthritis is a condition that can cause a plethora of symptoms, including deterioration of muscles and joints, a reduction of use in your main joints, and of course, severe pain.

Some cases of arthritis, like rheumatoid, can affect the immune system as well. There are constant and active studies on the conditions and your doctor knows the best treatment options for your specific situation.

Fortunately, on top of the modern medical treatment of arthritis, there are a few different things you can do daily to reduce and relieve the symptoms. Some studies have even shown that some of these all-natural treatments can even diminish symptoms of different types of arthritis!

In the following report, we will discuss 10 of the most widely used, all-natural forms of treatment for your arthritis symptoms.

Most of the following treatments can even be done in the comfort of your own home, and can be combined with current medical treatments you may be receiving.

Hopefully, with implementation you can begin to live a healthier and more pain-free life with arthritis.

Let's begin!

<u>Important Note:</u> It's important that you seek the advice and approval from your health care provider prior to making any drastic changes to your diet, exercise, or supplement intake.

Tip #1: Regular Exercise

Exercise is vital to keeping those joints and muscles elongated, warmed up, and moving. Make sure to always discuss your weight and exercise routine with your physician before following any workout plan.

Keep in mind that exercise doesn't have to mean 7 days at the gym pumping iron and running on treadmills. Regular movement, whether it's walking around your home or participating in aerobic classes at your gym, does wonders for arthritic pain.

In the past, it was thought that exercise made arthritis pain worse, but this has been shown to, not only be untrue, but quite the opposite. Daily workouts help to build and maintain a strong and healthy cardiovascular and muscular system.

Beyond the strengthening and stretching you get from exercise, maintaining a healthy weight contributes in many other ways as well, such as reducing the strain on muscles and joints. If you are overweight, it is important that you set goals with your physician to reach your optimal healthy weight and that you set yourself up for long-term success, rather than short-term results.

Laura Robbins, Senior Vice President of Education and Academic Affairs at the Hospital for Special Surgery in New York, says that for every pound you lose, you reduce the pressure on your knees by four pounds.

In fact, Roy Altman, MD, Professor of Medicine at the University of California, has seen symptoms of arthritis completely disappear from patients that have lost ten to twenty pounds of excess weight.

Along with the symptoms of arthritis, you will be improving your overall mental and physical well-being, helping to control other ailments your body may face as you age. A strong heart and a strong mind can do wonders for pain management!

Tip #2: Hot & Cold Treatments

One of the main natural treatments for arthritis include hot and cold treatments. There are several different types of arthritis so make sure to ask your doctor which will be better for your specific symptoms.

Cold Therapy helps to reduce joint swelling and inflammation. This type of treatment is most often recommended to rheumatoid arthritis sufferers, but can help others as well.

You can alternate hot and cold treatments as needed but always monitor how your skin reacts and adjust or discontinue as needed.

Cold treatments should be limited to 20-minute sessions. Here are several cold treatments used:

- Use a cloth covered bag of ice applied to the painful area.
- Submerge the joint in an ice bath.
  NOTE: *Check with a physician before submerging, especially if it is a large area of the body.*
- Simple cold packs kept in fridge or freezer, applied when needed.

Heat therapy is often good for all other types of arthritis, as well as, in conjunction with cold treatments. The heat relaxes your muscles and helps blood flow to the affected area.

Heat treatments should be monitored and adjusted depending upon your body's reaction.

Here are several heat treatments widely used by arthritis sufferers:

- Start your day with a hot bath or shower to get your blood flowing and joints relaxed.
- A warm paraffin wax to affected joints. (This can often be done by a professional to monitor wax temperature.)
- Apply a heating pad, heat pack, or other warm heat source to the affected joints.

Always make sure, when using heat therapy, to maintain a comfortable level of heat.

Hot tubs are also excellent ways to cover larger areas of the body, but always check with your physician first as they can be dangerous for those with certain health conditions.

Tip #3: Acupuncture

Acupuncture has been around for centuries and is an ancient Chinese Medicine. This process involves a medical professional trained in the art, inserting thin needles into specific pressure points on your body.

The focus of acupuncture is to reroute the energy stored behind your pain, and balance it throughout the body. It may sound gimmicky, but acupuncture is actually one of the most researched alternative therapies in the world, and is even recommended by the World Health Organization for a multitude of ailments.

Acupuncture is also one of the oldest pain remedies in history, and is completely natural. These tiny needles are stimulating the energy laid out in pathways across your body, called meridians. Studies have shown that acupuncture lowers the levels of inflammation inducing chemicals in the body.

Keep in mind that acupuncture cannot be safely administered by anyone except for a trained and certified acupuncturist.

The needles not only need to be placed in very specific spots connected to your specific ailments, but there is a rigorous hygienic process as well. Make sure to speak to your doctor, and get a referral if necessary, to find the right practitioner for you.

And don't worry, it may sound painful, but the needles are barely inserted into the skin, keeping the process relaxing and rejuvenating.

Tip #4: Omega-3 Fatty Acids

Omega-3 Fatty Acids have made the headlines in natural health for some time now, and for good reason. They are essential to a healthy and strong body. Omega-3 are good fats, ones you find mostly in plants and marine life. There are two main types of Omega-3's that are most commonly found in oily fish.

EPA (Eicosapentaenoic Acid)- EPA is the most well-known of the Omega-3's. It is a name arthritis sufferers want to remember. EPA not only helps to breakdown and synthesize those chemicals responsible for blood-clotting but it also helps dramatically with inflammation.

But where does EPA come from?

The simple answer to this is fish. Fish oil contains an abundance of EPA. The fish get this important Omega-3 from the algae that they eat. EPA fish oil is available in a variety of ways, but is easiest consumed through capsules sold at your local grocer or health food store.

DHA (Docosahexaenoic Acid)- DHA is another important Omega-3. DHA is a natural fatty acid abundant in the human body. It makes up the key parts of the retina in the eye, and part of the brain, the cerebral cortex.

The Cerebral Cortex, or grey matter, is responsible for intelligence, personality, motor function, organization, touch, sensory information processing, and language. These things are vital to your everyday existence and can play a huge part in pain management.

You can find Omega-3's in a variety of food, not just fish oil. These foods include nuts, cold-water fish like salmon and tuna, seeds, and other supplements.

In a 2015 study on the role of Omega-3's on inflammatory diseases, it is found that they can reduce symptoms of Rheumatoid and other arthritis symptoms.

Regardless of their pain management abilities, Omega-3 fatty acids should be a regular addition to your healthy and active lifestyle. Check with your physician to see which form of Omega-3's best fit your lifestyle.

Tip #5: Turmeric

Turmeric is nicknamed the *Golden Spice* and not just for its rich golden color. Turmeric studies are ongoing, but its health benefits seem to be growing by the day. This spice is found in many different curries and is harvested in India and Indonesia.

It's nothing new. Turmeric has been part of traditional medicine for centuries!

At the base of the healing properties of turmeric, it has been found to block the protein that causes inflammation. Because of these blocking abilities, turmeric has been found to ease the pain of inflammation just as well as some nonsteroidal anti-inflammatory drugs, or NASAIDs.

And it's all natural, which makes it even better.

The chemical in turmeric that does all the heavy lifting is called curcumin, and is the secret to its anti-inflammatory abilities.

While inflammation does play an important role in our bodies, blocking pathogens that could easily kill us, long term chronic inflammation like that observed in arthritis sufferers can be debilitating.

Inflammation is a complex process, but the curcumin in turmeric is an inflammation fighting bioactive substance that attacks the chronic inflammation on a molecular level.

On top of helping with your arthritic pain, curcumin has been shown to fight inflammation that also plays a major role in heart disease, cancer, Alzheimer's and many other conditions.

Turmeric can be taken in many ways from pills to the actual root. Why not add it to your favorite dish? On its own, turmeric has a very mild taste and can compliment almost any meal.

Tip #6: Massage Therapy

Massage therapy has long-term, lasting effects on pain management. The Arthritis Foundation has indicated that a regular massage to the muscles and joints helps to soothe the pain from arthritis.

If you've ever gotten a massage, you know that it can greatly increase your mood. This effect is because massages boost the levels of serotonin in your body, a chemical that contributes to happiness and well-being.

What you might not know is that massage therapy can also lower the body's production of cortisol, a stress inducing hormone that also helps the production of a neurotransmitter, Substance P. Substance P has a strong link to pain.

Several studies have been performed, most notably in 2013 by researchers at the Touch Research Institute, and 2015 by the

University of Miami School of Medicine. Both studies show that moderate touch massage therapy not only can reduce pain, but improve on grip, range of motion, and pressure.

Massages should be done by a licensed professional and is best performed by those with arthritis specialties. You can always let your therapist know of any sore areas to be avoided, and work with them to find the best pressure for your body.

Stiff muscles and joints are often exacerbated by stress and tension which we struggle to avoid when in pain so regular massages will help alleviate these issues.

So, lay back and relax, and let a professional massage therapist massage those aching joints and muscles! And don't be afraid to ask your specialist for at home massage techniques you can do yourself between sessions.

Tip #7: Aquatic Therapy

For years, it's been said that aquatic activity is one of the healthiest forms of exercise that a person can participate in. It is beneficial for all types of people, but especially those with arthritis.

What makes aquatic activity so useful when managing pain associated with arthritis?

Water provides natural resistance, which in turn intensifies the exercises you are performing.

At the same time, water has something that regular exercise does not, *buoyancy*. That tendency for your bodies to float in water helps to support your body weight, thus reducing the pressure on your joints. Less pressure means less inflammation, and less inflammation leads to less pain.

Pain isn't the only thing that aquatic therapy helps though. The natural intensity of your movements helps to reduce body fat, improves your coordination, your range of motion, and has a positive effect on serotonin levels in the brain. Again, a less stressed body leads to less stress on joints and bones.

A 2015 study by the University of Utah showed that aquatic exercise for pain management in adults, especially those over 65, can vastly improve mobility and pain. While the pain reduction was short term, aquatic therapy shows to be an excellent alternative to pain medication for quick relief.

You can find on-going relief with aquatic therapy by performing up to an hour of aquatic exercise three times a week. So, not only will you reduce or maintain your weight, but you will find a mood stimulating and pain reducing activity to help with your symptoms of arthritis.

Tip #8: Tai Chi

Tai Chi can be incorporated into your daily exercise routine. The perfect type of exercise for people with arthritis is that in which improves muscular strength, improves fitness, and builds on flexibility. Tai Chi does all these things through a low impact exercise routine.

Tai Chi is a slow moving, low-impact, easy form of martial arts. It's appropriate for anyone that can move freely. The art is composed of a series of slow and gentle movements, all easily modified for those with sore and stiff joints.

Tai Chi has also been shown to help with muscle strength, flexibility, and balance.

In 2013, researchers China reviewed 7 different studies on Tai Chi in reference to arthritis.

They performed a meta-analysis to assess the effectiveness of Tai Chi exercise for pain, stiffness, and physical function. In conclusion, they stated that a 12-week course can be beneficial to arthritis sufferers when it comes to reducing pain, reducing stiffness of joints and muscles, and increasing their physical functionality.

When muscles are strong, they help to protect the joints, reducing pain. Flexibility keeps those joints loose and reduces stiffness. And an increase in balance can help to reduce the number of falls arthritis sufferers face. All of these things are results of a regular Tai Chi workout.

Tai Chi classes can be found both privately through martial arts institutions and through public programs.

Many senior facilities also offer Tai Chi several times a week. Even those bound to wheelchairs can find benefits from modified movements.

Tip #9: Yoga

Yoga is a 5,000-year-old practice, originated in ancient India, and spread through the world. There are many different forms of yoga that include poses, breathing techniques, and meditation.

It has the ability to boost both mental and physical health of its practitioners.

Yoga is a very gentle exercise, a way to reduce the tension in joints and muscles, build muscle tone, and increase flexibility.

That muscle strength can also help to improve balance, especially important to those with arthritis. Yoga is low-impact and enjoyable in nature, making it easy to practice on a regular basis.

Some of Yoga's many benefits include:

- Adds variety to your exercise routine.

- Strengthening to improve physical functionality.
- Improvement in flexibility which reduces inflammation and stiffness.
- Weight loss can be a benefit of Yoga done correctly and in conjunction with a healthy diet.
- Strengthening of the mind-body connection which allows for better balance and understanding of the pains and stiffness you feel on a regular basis.

As with all exercise routines, make sure to check with your physician before starting any regiment. If you are new to Yoga, it is best to seek instruction.

Yoga facilities have grown widely across the world, and you can do both private and group classes.

Tip #10: Meditation

Meditation is a practice you can do anytime, anywhere. One of the biggest parts of meditation is practicing **mindfulness**.

When you practice mindfulness meditation, you are focusing all of your attention on the feelings and sensations that your body is experiencing in that present moment.

There is a program available to you that focuses solely on this form of meditation. It is called Mindfulness-Based Stress Reduction, or MBSR.

MBSR is used to help you manage both pain and stress. These two negative attributes of arthritis are not only hard to deal with, but also contribute to a diminished immune system.

A healthy immune system is vital to fighting off disease as well as keeping your body as pain-free and relaxed as possible.

In 2014, researchers performed a study on the effectiveness of MBSR with people suffering from rheumatoid arthritis. It was found that those that completed the eight week sessions reported a reduction in pain, stiffness, and tender and swollen joints.

It is amazing what the mind can do, and this type of program can be easily incorporated into your daily routine without putting aside a ton of extra time or effort.

Final Words

Arthritis is something that takes a toll on not just the body, but the mind as well. Luckily, as you've seen in this report, there are a multitude of all-natural and homeopathic routines that you can incorporate into your daily life to help reduce your pain and improve the quality of your life.

Through regular exercise and weight management you can help your body deal with the degenerative effects of arthritis, while also improving your health and wellness.

Adding to that, increasing your amount of Omega-3, adding a little turmeric into your weekly routine, and engaging in one or more of the low-impact therapies and exercises available, you could finally find a natural relief to your aches and pains!

This report in no way states that you should forgo the treatment regimen set up between you and your doctor, but adding these to your day-to-day life will help to relieve that in which medications do not.

And you never know, you may be able to reduce the amount of pain medications you take and replace them with natural and effective methods of pain management. ☺

We wish you the very best on your new journey toward a stronger, more flexible, and pain free future!

Resources

Here are links to a few resources that I believe will help you:

Fish Oils and Omega-3:

https://www.medicalnewstoday.com/articles/40253#what_are_omega_3_fatty_acids

Lutein Skincare Benefits: 13 Natural Remedies for Arthritis

https://www.health.com/condition/osteoarthritis/13-natural-remedies-for-arthritis

Relief from Arthritis: Natural Relief Strategies

https://www.healthline.com/health/osteoarthritis/arthritis-natural-relief

Home Remedies:

https://www.medicalnewstoday.com/articles/324446

The Best Home Remedies for Arthritis

Tai Chi and Arthritis:

https://journals.plos.org/plosone/article?id=10.1371/journal.pon e.0061672

Yoga Benefits:

https://www.arthritis.org/health-wellness/healthy-living/physical- activity/yoga/yoga-benefits-for-arthritis

www.ingramcontent.com/pod-product-compliance
Lightning Source LLC
Chambersburg PA
CBHW042013110726
48006CB00004B/1069